ENDORSEMENTS

Lillian Baker has written a must-read about God's redeeming love—a transformative guide filled with biblical truth to direct you on your path of spiritual strength. *Built to Last* is for the one who has lost hope, the people pleaser, the broken-hearted, the new believer, or someone firm in their walk who yearns for a fresh perspective. I wish I had something like this as a youth. Truly impactful—so much truth into words.

Elissia Forty LSW

Built to Last is a highly engaging book and an enjoyable read! The author is real and raw right up front, which causes the reader to let their guard down. The chapter on "Serving Beyond Self" was brutally honest and really leaves you thinking. She walked the wayward path that many of us do and demonstrates how to overcome by example. And if she can change, it feels manageable for us to change. It's like you have your very own Spiritual Life Coach right by your side rooting you on!

Linda Slomin, MA, LPC
Author of *The Very Sensitive Princess*

Built to Last is a must read for anyone who needs to plug into empowerment and walk into their purpose.

L. Michelle Smith, LMS, Author
Call and Response: 10 Leadership Lessons from the Black Church

This incredible and powerful book is so timely as it is written to a world that needs to be encouraged to fight the good fight. Lillian's real life, saturated with the presence of God, helped her to persevere and push through difficult times. This book will challenge you, inspire you, it'll make you cry and make you laugh, but at the end of the day, this book will give you the tools to live the abundant life. A great read that will launch you to walk and live in victory!

Rev. Tony Cotto
Lead Pastor, Chestnut A/G Church

Built to Last by Lillian Baker is an excellent study guide for both group and individual study. Through honest personal testimonies of the adversities she faced from childhood to young adulthood, and even health challenges, Baker shares encouraging lessons learned and how her relationship with Jesus helped her go from someone with a low self-esteem to now someone who is a life coach and encourages others to grow deeper in their faith. Each chapter offers life lessons rooted in God's Word, making the book both practical and encouraging. I especially appreciated the pre- and post-session assessments as well as the "notes" sections, which provide a meaningful way to reflect on and measure spiritual growth. This book is a valuable resource for anyone seeking to grow in their faith through strong foundational principals found in God's Word.

Pastor Ken and Tiffany Corson
Fairton Christian Center

In *Built to Last: A Spiritual Guide for Strength, Purpose, and Impact,* Lillian Baker delivers a profound and practical blueprint for living a life rooted in faith, resilience, and purpose. A must read as her words remind us that true impact is forged not in fleeting moments, but in the steady strength of a spirit anchored in God.

Dr. Gary L. Wilder, DMin.
Retired U.S. Marine Corps Master Sergeant
Author of *One Degree: Unleashing Your Focus*
Founder & CEO, Directional Moments Coaching

BUILT TO LAST

A Spiritual Training Guide for Strength, Purpose, and Impact

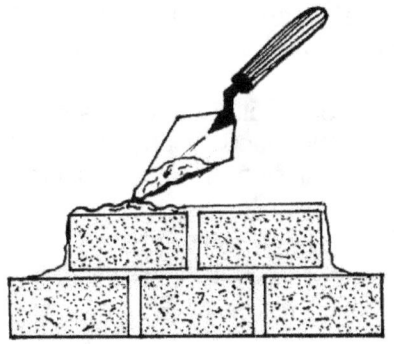

LILLIAN BAKER

Pageant Wagon Publishing
Vineland, NJ

Built to Last: A Spiritual Training Guide for Strength, Purpose, and Impact
Copyright ©2025 Lillian Baker

ISBN: 978-1-7360080-8-9

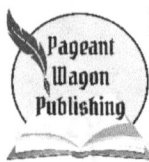

Editor: Kathryn Ross
Published by Pageant Wagon Publishing
Pageant Wagon Productions LLC
Interior Art by Stacy Lee Flury

Copyright 2025 by Lillian Baker. All Rights Reserved. No part of this publication may be reproduced, stored in a retrieval system, or transmitted in any form or by any means without prior permission in writing from the author, with the exception of brief excerpts in magazine articles or reviews, citing the author, in accordance with the Fair Use Act.

Unless otherwise noted, all Scriptures are referenced from the New King James Version®. Copyright © 1982 by Thomas Nelson. Used by permission. All rights reserved.

The ESV® Bible (The Holy Bible, English Standard Version®), © 2001 by Crossway, a publishing ministry of Good News Publishers. ESV Text Edition: 2025.

Holy Bible, New International Version®, NIV® Copyright ©1973, 1978, 1984, 2011 by Biblica, Inc.® Used by permission. All rights reserved worldwide.

DEDICATION

To my Lord and Savior, Jesus Christ,
all glory belongs to You. Thank you for your mercy
and grace. You are my foundation, my healer, and the
builder of my life. Without Your grace,
these words would have no meaning.

To my husband, Paul,
thank you for walking beside me with patience, love,
and unwavering support. Your encouragement has
been the quiet strength behind my steps,
and your faith in me has given me courage and
confidence when I needed it most.

To the readers of this book,
thank you for choosing to journey with me through
these pages. This book is for you who long for a
strong foundation, even when life feels uncertain
or imperfect. May you be reminded that God does not
ask for perfection, only alignment with His truth.
Strength comes not from flawlessness, but
from building your life on the solid ground of Christ.

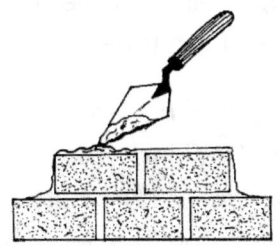

ACKNOWLEDGEMENTS

First, all glory and gratitude to God—my firm foundation and faithful guide. Every page of this book was built through His grace, wisdom, and strength.

Paul, I am deeply grateful for your encouragement throughout this process. Your faith in me has been a reminder that I never walk alone, and your support gave me the strength to see this book to completion.
Angel, Joshua, Christina, and Rebekah—thank you for celebrating this milestone with me and for being proud of the dreams I've pursued.

To my church family and friends who believed in the message before it had a cover—your encouragement helped me keep building.

A special thank you to those whose voices spoke truth and healing into my life, especially Pam, who welcomed me into a divorce support group during a season when I needed hope most. I may not remember every exact detail, but I will never forget the worth and healing spoken over me there. It restored my hope and remained instrumental in shaping the woman I am today.

To Kathryn Ross, my patient and persistent editor, who never stopped asking when I would finally write this book—thank you. When I stepped out in faith to begin, you guided me through the process with wisdom, grace, and steady encouragement. Your belief in me helped bring this vision to life.

To the communities, coaches, and leaders who poured into me, and to the readers who will carry these words into your own journeys—you are all part of these pages.

May this book remind you, as it has reminded me, that when we build our lives on Christ the Solid Rock, we are truly built to last.

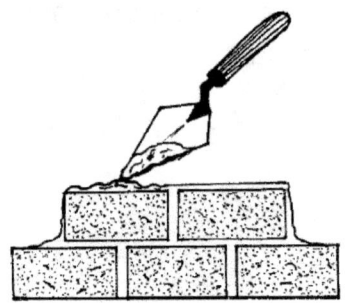

TABLE OF CONTENTS

Introduction ~ Page 1

Pre-Session Assessment ~ Page 5

Session 1: The Crucible of Childhood
~ Page 7 ~

Session 2: Spoken Words Breed Rooted Thoughts
~ Page 18 ~

Session 3: Boundaries: Guardrails of Grace
~ Page 31 ~

Session 4: Serving Beyond Self
~ Page 42 ~

Session 5: Everyday Habits—Eternal Impact
~ Page 59 ~

Session 6: Vision Born from Purpose
~ Page 72 ~

Session 7: A Grateful Heart
~ Page 84 ~

Post-Session Assessment ~ Page 94

Final Blessing ~ Page 98

About the Author ~ Page 99

About Pageant Wagon Publishing ~ Page 100

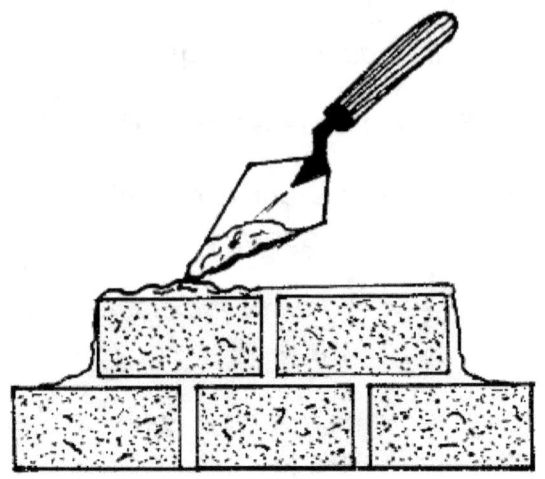

Everyone who comes to Me and hears My words and does them, I will show you what he is like: he is like a man building a house, who dug deep and laid the foundation on the rock. And when a flood arose, the stream broke against that house and could not shake it, because it had been well built.

Luke 6:47–48 ESV

INTRODUCTION

Throughout my life's journey, I have encountered many storms—some I created myself, and others arrived uninvited. In those times, I found myself questioning God, wondering if I had what it took to withstand the weight of it all. Even with faith in my heart, I wrestled with feelings of inadequacy and the lie that I was undeserving of God's grace because of my flaws.

But in my late twenties, something shifted. I made a conscious decision to turn fully to God—not just when it was convenient, but in *every* situation. I began to seek His guidance like a builder leaning on a blueprint, trusting Him to lead me through life's construction zone.

I learned to pause before every crossroad, to consider each step carefully. I could isolate and remain in my unfinished state, or I could submit to the Master Builder, allowing Him to teach and shape me through each trial. I chose the latter. With every storm I faced, I leaned harder into Him, determined to let His Word become the bedrock of my life.

God helped me stand strong—not by removing the trials, but by reinforcing my spiritual structure. Like building a tower that won't topple in the wind, I had to dig deep and reinforce the foundation. It took soul-level excavation, consistent surrender, and daily alignment with His truth. This was not a quick build,

Introduction

but a lifelong process of constructing something sturdy and lasting.

If you've ever wrestled with feelings of uncertainty, weariness, or weakness, know this: You are not alone. God invites *all* of us to be built up—to become strong and unshakable through Him. In a world of shifting ground and constant distractions, having a well-anchored mind and spirit is essential. The strength to withstand life's storms isn't found in outer displays, but in the inner framework of our lives—our thoughts, our beliefs, and our trust in God.

Though no metaphor is perfect, the idea of constructing a solid structure is one we can all understand. Just as a sturdy building requires the right materials and a strong foundation, so does a spiritually resilient life. Our faith becomes unshakable when we invest in spiritual disciplines that act as bricks and beams, aligning us with God's design.

This study guide is your blueprint for building a faith that lasts. Together, we'll lay essential cornerstones—reading and meditating on Scripture, worship, prayer, gratitude, and aligning your thoughts and words with God's truth. Each of these will serve as vital building blocks in your spiritual structure, helping you withstand life's pressures with grace and stability.

This journey is not about perfection. It's about construction—letting the Holy Spirit work in you to create something enduring. With each lesson, you'll

Introduction

take practical steps toward building up your faith, reinforcing your mind, and anchoring your life on God's promises.

You are not building alone. *Built to Last: A Spiritual Training Guide for Strength, Purpose, and Impact* is your companion on this sacred project.

Reinforcing your mind and spirit isn't just about surviving hard times—it's about *thriving* in every season through the power of Christ. Let's begin this building process together, supporting one another as we rise stronger, brick by brick.

Jesus reminds us in John 16:33, *"I have told you these things, so that in me you may have peace. In this world you will have trouble. But take heart! I have overcome the world."*

We have a choice: to remain in spiritual ruins or rise up and be built into something beautiful. You are invited to take part in a holy construction project—one that will strengthen not only your life but your legacy. As your spiritual coach, I'll walk with you step by step as we:

- Assess the current condition of your foundation.
- Identify areas that need repair, reinforcement, or rebuilding.
- Embrace intentional practices that strengthen your inner structure.
- Discover and build toward God's unique assignment for your life.

Introduction

How to Use This Book

This is not just a study—it's a hands-on building project. *Built to Last* is interactive by design, calling you to reflect, respond, and apply. You won't simply read and move on; you'll engage with God, examine your heart, and take action.

To make the most of this journey, invest in a journal, or you may opt to use the "Notes" section at the end of each session chapter. Pair it with your favorite pen and treat these as tools for spiritual construction. This will be how you pour out your thoughts, prayers, blueprints, and building progress.

Find a quiet space—your construction zone—where you can meet with God consistently. As you work through each session, complete the building practices, reflect prayerfully, and jot down what the Lord reveals as you reflect on the *Cornerstones of Growth* sections. Over time, your notes will become a beautiful testimony of the foundation you're laying and the tower God is raising in and through you.

This book is more than words on a page—it's a call to build. To construct a faith that holds steady through every season. To rise, unshaken, on the rock that never crumbles. Are you ready to begin? Let's build—together.

Lillian Baker

October 2025

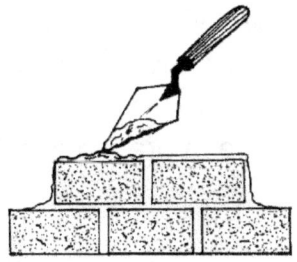

Pre-Assessment
Where Are You Now in Your Spiritual Health Journey?

Complete this personal inventory before starting *Built to Last*. This is not a test. It's an honest snapshot of where you are spiritually right now.

Use your journal to record your answers and reflections. Return to review your answers in comparison to the *Post-Assessment* at the end of the book to see how far you've come.

For each question below, rate yourself on a scale from 1 to 5:
1 = Not at all   2 = Rarely   3 = Sometimes
4 = Often   5 = Consistently

Self-Reflection & Spiritual Awareness
I take time to reflect on my life and my walk with God.
Answer: _____

Pre-Assessment

I seek God's perspective on my circumstances rather than reacting based on my emotions. Answer: _____

I regularly spend time in prayer and the Word of God. Answer: _____

Identifying Areas for Growth

I am aware of the spiritual areas in my life that need strengthening. Answer: _____

I take intentional steps to renew my mind and align my thoughts with God's truth. Answer: _____

I recognize and challenge negative thoughts that do not align with God's promises. Answer: _____

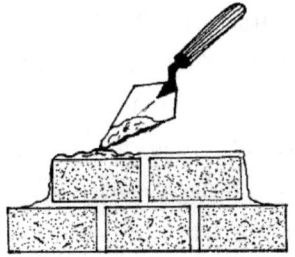

Session 1
The Crucible of Childhood

My childhood unfolded in the gritty streets of the Gowanus Projects in Brooklyn, New York where I learned to navigate a world of conflicting emotions.

The pounding thump-thump-thump, then swish-cheer, with shouts of obscenities following and back to thump-thump-thump, rose up from the concrete court below my 4th floor apartment building as I watched from a window. Basketball looked like fun.

"Can't I go out and play, too, Mom?"

"No," Mom replied firmly. "Too dangerous outside these days. Find something inside to play with."

Perhaps this is where my interest in human behavior began. I entertained myself inside by observing people of all kinds outside and made up stories in my head about them.

Session 1: The Crucible of Childhood

Born into a Hispanic family of five, I was right smack in the middle of three older brothers and one younger sister. My parents, both factory workers, labored tirelessly to provide for us. They loved us dearly and were strict, devout Christians. But even though I felt the warmth of their consistent love and care, a dark secret lurked in the shadows that would shape my life for years to come.

As a latch-key child, I returned home from school many days to an empty apartment. My only companions were the flickering images on the television and the well-worn pages of books. I cherished them as my escape—a refuge from the harsh realities of the outside world.

And I desperately needed a place of refuge in those days.

A family friend from our church, whom I trusted and looked to as a protector, often met me on my walk home from school and joined me with happy chatter. But there were times he fell into step beside me that his hand brushed up against mine. It felt cold and rough—a creepy sensation. This happened more times than not after a while, and I came to fear the end of the school day because he might appear again.

Eventually, I devised an escape plan—run as fast as possible to get ahead of him on the way so he would miss me. Sometimes I was successful. Other times he found me and stopped me in my tracks to

Session 1: The Crucible of Childhood

walk at pace with him. His presence alarmed me but due to my upbringing and family culture, I was taught to respect my elders and allowed him into my personal space.

Normally, he seemed to have a lot to say as we walked on the street. But once we started up the four flights of the stairwell, we climbed in silence. An eerie, uncomfortable silence that came with a sense of foreboding. He'd leave me at the top of the stairwell, and I felt like a prisoner let loose. Once on the other side of the door to the fourth-floor hallway, I breathed a sigh of relief. Yet—felt jittery inside all the same.

The first time he molested me with unwelcome touch, I was about seven or eight years old. The memory of my innocence stolen was soul-imbedded with a host of associated imagery: the smell of damp concrete and old cigarettes, the cool, rough surface of the cinder block wall scraping against my skin. A dull, reddish-brown metal handrail loomed in the corner of my vision, its paint chipped and peeling like old wounds. I focused on it, on the cracks in the wall, on anything but what was happening to me.

I didn't realize it at the time, but that day something inside of me shifted. I would never be the same. After that first encounter, it was as though he assumed he had full permission to repeat the offense. And with each offense, I withdrew more and more—dying a little on the inside. Laying a foundation for vain attempts at self-preservation. Like the cracked cinder

Session 1: The Crucible of Childhood

block walls of the stairwell, invisible bricks stacked up and mortared themselves on top of that foundation and around my heart. Cemented into my child's psyche, this cinder block wall was my only recourse to protect myself from anyone trying to share personal space with me again. I wouldn't even realize I had built such walls until years later.

His actions repulsed me, but it was easier to stay silent because I didn't know how to address what had happened to me. The episodes of molestation continued for a while until just like that—he was gone. Vanished without a trace. I never saw him again. To this day I have no idea what became of him. He never came to visit my parents, and they never mentioned or talked about him again.

Through this experience at such an early and impressionable age, I learned to hold my emotions and my voice in. I learned how to be two people. At church and school, I was the good girl—the one who followed the rules, never talked back, and made life easy for the adults around her.

But after school, I found myself drawn to other kids who felt like me: misfits, kids who didn't fit neatly into the expectations of home, church, or school. With them, I could let loose—at least a version of myself could let loose. I learned to smoke and play hooky from school, experimenting with inappropriate ways to express myself. But none of it felt like me. The real

Session 1: The Crucible of Childhood

me in the deepest places of my being. It was just another mask. Another role to play.

Along the way, as I grew in mask-making, I mastered the art of reading a room and molding myself accordingly. If I couldn't take up space with my voice, I would make myself useful in other ways, adopting a promiscuous lifestyle. The only problem was that those ways weren't healthy. Over time, I became an introvert—not because I disliked people, but because I believed the world around me taught me that my words were not of any value. Silence became my way of life. The cracked cinder block wall climbed higher and higher, fortified as each youthful year passed.

By the time I reached adulthood, I no longer knew who I really was. I sought validation in work, relationships, and achievements, and hoped someone would finally see me. The real me.

But no matter how much I accomplished, emptiness remained. My lack of personal identity shaped my thoughts, actions, and interactions—through two divorces, childbearing, and far too many dead ends in life.

One day, though, I met someone different. A soft-spoken, slender blonde lady with a pretty face and kind demeanor befriended me when I visited her church after my second divorce. She invited me to the divorce support group that she led. Her non-judgmental way disarmed me, and I felt a cinder block

Session 1: The Crucible of Childhood

topple. She truly listened and somehow heard my heart. The real me in that deep, walled place.

More cinder blocks crumbled. I stood on the threshold of healing.

My new friend became a mentor who spoke words of worth over me. And though I had been a church goer all my life, she introduced me to the Jesus who lives outside of religion and desires a true, living relationship with . . . ME!

I had never known Jesus in that way. I knew He was God's holy Son who came into the earth, which we celebrated at Christmas with presents under a tree. He saved us from our sin by His death on the cross and resurrection, which was part of why I got an Easter basket in the spring.

As a little girl, that was just the way it was, but I understood nothing beyond those words at face value and ritual traditions surrounding each holiday. No depth of meaning to me on a personal level. On a spiritual level.

But something in the way my kind friend explained who Jesus was opened my soul to want to know more and to truly understand this great love for me that she said He had. When I allowed the possibility that Jesus truly was alive and could speak directly to me—and knew me—I heard Him whisper to my heart, *You are seen. You are loved. You have a voice.*

Session 1: The Crucible of Childhood

And the walls came tumbling down! The little, wounded girl on the other side of those walls was free. Jesus loved ME! My spirit came alive, and I was born again.

It wasn't easy to unlearn years of silence and pent-up behaviors, let alone a whole lot of empty theology. But I took a step of faith. Then another. Then another. I journaled my thoughts. I spoke up in meetings. I prayed with confidence. I sought the Lord with all of my soul and He found me every time I reached out for Him. I was transformed!

Scripture reveals that through faith in Jesus Christ, we become new creations: *"Therefore, if anyone is in Christ, he is a new creation; old things have passed away; behold, all things have become new"* 2 Corinthians 5:17.

This transformation is not merely superficial; it signifies a profound change in our very essence. We become children of God, chosen and dearly loved: *"But you are a chosen generation, a royal priesthood, a holy nation, His own special people, that you may proclaim the praises of Him who called you out of darkness into His marvelous light."* 1 Peter 2:9.

Understanding my identity in Christ opened the door to experience true forgiveness. The results of the fall of Adam are reversed in the earth by the work of Jesus on the cross. Through Jesus' sacrifice, I received redemption and the complete forgiveness of

Session 1: The Crucible of Childhood

my sins: *"In Him we have redemption through His blood, the forgiveness of sins, according to the riches of His grace."* Ephesians 1:7.

This forgiveness is not earned by our efforts but is a gift of grace—the unmerited favor of God towards us who believe—underscoring the depth of God's love for us. Embracing God's forgiveness transformed my heart and enabled me to extend forgiveness to the man who wronged me, through the redeeming power of Jesus within me.

Jesus teaches us to forgive others as He has also forgiven us. This act of forgiving others is not only a reflection of our obedience to Christ but also a pathway to personal freedom and healing. True transformation arises from an authentic, saving relationship with Jesus Christ, where His presence empowers us to live out our faith—what we believe—dynamically.

The journey from confronting lies to embracing the truth of our identity in Christ is transformative. It liberates us from past hurts and empowers us to forgive others, reflecting the forgiveness we have received. This new life is marked by a vibrant relationship with God, moving beyond mere religious practices into the fullness of His love and purpose for us.

My day of transformation and healing came when I looked in the mirror and saw someone I recognized—Me. Not the girl who was taken advantage of. Not the

Session 1: The Crucible of Childhood

girl shaped by quiet expectations or unhealthy escapes. But the woman God created me to be. I have a voice, and I now know how to use it.

Cornerstones of Growth

- **Personal Reflection:** Can you identify any lies you've believed about yourself that contradicts God's Word? How does embracing your identity in Christ challenge those falsehoods?

- **Forgiveness Journey:** Reflect on a time when you found it difficult to forgive someone. How does understanding God's forgiveness toward you influence your ability to forgive others?

- **Authentic Faith:** In what ways can you cultivate a deeper, more authentic relationship with God, moving beyond routine religious practices?

NOTES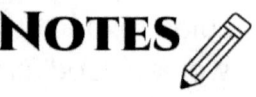

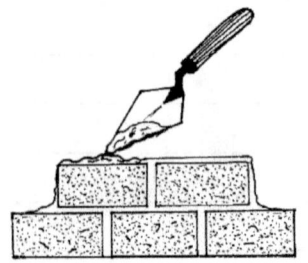

Session 2
Spoken Words Breed Rooted Thoughts

I was a young girl when I first heard the words.

"Left-handed people don't go to heaven," my mother said as she watched me struggling to cut a piece of meat at the dinner table.

I froze, my small fingers gripping the fork awkwardly. "What?" I asked, looking up at her.

She chuckled, shaking her head. "You do everything backwards. I don't know what we're going to do with you." She said, taking the utensils from my hands and placing them in the "right" position. "Left-handed people . . . well, they just don't go to heaven."

I was just a child, but that single phrase—spoken so many times—took root in my mind and began to grow. *If I wasn't going to heaven anyway, why even try to be good? Why should I seek a God who had already rejected me?*

Session 2: Spoken Words Breed Rooted Thoughts

The older I got, the more my mother tried to help me "fit" into a right-handed world. She never did it with malice. I believe she thought she was doing what was best for me—helping me navigate life more easily.

One of my clearest memories is of when I was old enough to start ironing. I was excited to learn and eager to do something that made me feel grown-up. I grabbed the iron with my left hand, but before I could press it onto the fabric, my mother stopped me.

"No, no, use your right hand," she said, gently guiding my left hand away and placing the iron in my right.

"But this feels weird," I protested, trying to adjust my grip.

"You'll get used to it," she assured me. "It'll be easier in the long run. Trust me, the world is made for right-handed people."

I sighed and tried again, but the movement felt unnatural. The iron felt heavier, my strokes uneven. The fabric bunched up under the weight of my awkward pressing.

"Like this," my mother said, demonstrating with smooth, confident motions. "See? You don't want to leave wrinkles. Keep the iron steady."

I tried to mimic her movements, but my right hand lacked the coordination of my left. The task that had

Session 2: Spoken Words Breed Rooted Thoughts

felt exciting moments ago now felt frustrating and tedious.

I didn't understand her reasoning at the time, but I obeyed. And after enough practice, the awkwardness faded. To this day, ironing is one of the very few things I still do with my right hand.

At the time, I didn't think much about it. But as I reflect now, I realize how easily these repeated messages—even spoken with good intentions—shaped my life as I grew older. Just as I learned to iron with my right hand despite being left-handed, I also unknowingly trained my mind to believe something that wasn't true: *Somehow, I was less acceptable because of the way I was made.*

Looking back, I can see how the enemy used those words to create a false belief system in my young heart. The battlefield of the mind is real, and the words spoken over us—whether intentional or not—can shape our thoughts, our actions, and even our faith. Proverbs 18:21 says, *"Death and life are in the power of the tongue, and those who love it will eat its fruit."*

I had unknowingly absorbed the fruit of careless words, and their seeds had taken deep root in my thinking, influencing the way I saw myself and my purpose.

But unfortunately, it doesn't stop with us. It's like a domino effect. If we never learn to take our thoughts

Session 2: Spoken Words Breed Rooted Thoughts

captive and watch what we say to others, we risk wasting the lives of the people God has placed in our sphere of influence.

Our thoughts shape our actions, and our actions shape our behavior, sending ripples into eternity. When we shut down under the weight of negative thinking, entire generations of kingdom builders may never be impacted as God intended. The enemy knows this well, and nothing pleases him more than seeing us stuck—paralyzed by doubt, distracted by lies, and spinning in place instead of moving forward in God's purpose.

This is his strategy. The battle begins in your mind, so never underestimate the power of your thoughts.

But God, in His grace, doesn't leave us trapped in lies. His truth uproots every deception. Romans 12:2 reminds us, *"And do not be conformed to this world, but be transformed by the renewing of your mind, that you may prove what is that good and acceptable and perfect will of God."*

My transformation didn't happen overnight. It took a long time to replace the lies with God's truth.

The truth is my left-handedness was never a flaw in God's eyes. He designed me with intention and purpose; no detail was a mistake. Psalm 139:13-14 says, *"For You formed my inward parts; You covered me in my mother's womb. I praise You, for I am*

Session 2: Spoken Words Breed Rooted Thoughts

fearfully and wonderfully made; marvelous are Your works, and that my soul knows very well."

This battle isn't unique to me. Many of us believe lies spoken over us—words from parents, teachers, friends, or even our self-doubt. We carry them for years, allowing them to define our identity and relationship with God. But God invites us to break free. His Word has the power to demolish every false stronghold.

The enemy wants to keep us bound by false narratives, but God calls us to freedom. The process of breaking free begins with identifying the lies, rejecting them, replacing them with the truth of God's Word, and renewing our minds daily. Let's break these down:

1. Recognize the Lie

We cannot fight what we do not identify. Many of us walk around with beliefs that limit our faith and distort our view of God, but we don't even realize it. Ask the Holy Spirit to reveal any lie you have believed about yourself. Psalm 139:23-24 says, *"Search me, O God, and know my heart; Try me, and know my anxieties; And see if there is any wicked way in me, And lead me in the way everlasting."*

Sometimes the most damaging lies are the ones spoken over us by family, teachers, friends, or even society. Words have power, and if we're not careful, we can internalize false identities that were never God's truth for us.

Session 2: Spoken Words Breed Rooted Thoughts

2. Reject the Lie

Not only do you need to recognize the lie, but you must also reject it. Lies may seem harmless or even comforting in the moment, but like empty calories, they weaken your spiritual core over time. If we let them settle in our minds, they distort our identity, weaken our faith, and keep us from living in the fullness of God's truth.

2 Corinthians 10:5 reminds *"casting down arguments and every high thing that exalts itself against the knowledge of God, bringing every thought into captivity to the obedience of Christ,"*

That means we don't passively accept every thought that enters our minds. Instead, we hold it up to the light of God's Word and ask: **Is this true? Does this align with what God says about me?**

If the answer is no, we must reject it—just as we would reject something toxic or spoiled that could damage our health.

You wouldn't build your body on spoiled food—and you shouldn't build your identity on toxic thoughts. Lies corrode your foundation. Truth reinforces it.

3. Replace It with Truth

Rejecting a lie isn't enough—you have to replace it with something stronger. Your mind, like your body, needs real nourishment to thrive. The truth of God's Word is what gives your spirit strength and stability.

Session 2: Spoken Words Breed Rooted Thoughts

If you remove what's harmful but don't refill with what's true, you'll still be left vulnerable. Our souls were created to be filled—so we must be intentional about filling them with what is good. Paul says in Philippians 4:8, *"Finally, brethren, whatever things are true, whatever things are noble, whatever things are just, whatever things are pure, whatever things are lovely, whatever things are of good report, if there is any virtue and if there is anything praiseworthy—meditate on these things."*

God's Word is the foundation your soul craves. Jesus said in Matthew 4:4, *"But He answered and said, 'It is written, 'Man shall not live by bread alone, but by every word that proceeds from the mouth of God.'"*

When a lie tries to take root in your mind, don't just push it aside—actively replace it with truth.
- If you believed the lie that you're not good enough, declare Psalm 139:14, *"I am fearfully and wonderfully made."*
- If you've struggled with the thought that God has abandoned you, stand on Deuteronomy 31:6, *"...for the Lord your God, He is the One who goes with you. He will not leave you nor forsake you."*

4. Renew the Mind Daily

Replacing lies with truth is a choice we must make—but it doesn't stop there.

Session 2: Spoken Words Breed Rooted Thoughts

Transformation happens through daily renewal. Just like a strong structure needs ongoing care, a spiritually strong life requires a consistent return to God's Word. The lies we've believed won't disappear overnight, and the enemy will always try to plant new ones.

We must make a habit of meditating on truth, speaking it, and building our inner world on it daily. Romans 12:2 reminds us, "*And do not be conformed to this world, but be transformed by the renewing of your mind, that you may prove what is that good and acceptable and perfect will of God.*"

Just like one brick doesn't make a whole wall, one Scripture reading doesn't build a lasting foundation. Daily renewal is what strengthens and transforms us over time.

5. Speak Life

What you build in your mind shapes you—but what you speak reinforces it. Proverbs 18:21 says, *"Death and life are in the power of the tongue."*

The words you speak can build up or tear down, strengthen faith or fuel doubt. Jesus set the example. When He was tempted in the wilderness, He didn't just think the truth—He spoke it aloud (Matthew 4:1–11). "It is written," He said again and again. If Jesus needed to speak the truth to defeat lies, how much more do we?

Session 2: Spoken Words Breed Rooted Thoughts

When I finally understood that being left-handed had nothing to do with my salvation, I had to retrain my mind to accept God's grace. But the real shift came when I spoke Ephesians 2:8-9 truth over myself, "I am saved by grace, not by works. God loves me completely, not because of what I do, but because of who He is."

Speaking the truth out loud reinforced what I was learning internally and helped me break from the lie.

A practical way to do this is through declarations—intentional statements of truth based on Scripture:
- Instead of saying, "I'm not good enough," speak Psalm 139:14, *"I am fearfully and wonderfully made."*
- Instead of saying, "I'll never be free from this struggle," declare John 8:36, *"Therefore if the Son makes you free, you shall be free indeed."*

Speaking life is a discipline that strengthens your faith and renews your foundation. Just as daily renewal builds internal strength, daily declarations bring breakthrough.

What you speak today can shape how you live tomorrow.

There was a time when I allowed false words to define me. But now I walk in the truth that I am loved, chosen, and accepted by God. I no longer believe the lie that I was rejected before I even had a chance.

Session 2: Spoken Words Breed Rooted Thoughts

Instead, I know that God formed me with care and that His plans for me are good.

The words spoken over us can shape our destiny—but only if we let them. Never forget: You are not a prisoner of your thoughts. You have the power to choose.

Spiritual strength is built one decision at a time. Keep stepping into freedom.

Cornerstones of Growth

1. Rewrite the Narrative:
    - ✓ Write down a negative phrase or lie you've believed about yourself.
    - ✓ Find a scripture that speaks the opposite truth.
    - ✓ Declare that truth daily.
    - ✓ Practice speaking life over yourself and others.
    - ✓ When a lie tries to take root in your mind, don't just push it aside—actively replace it with truth:
        - If you believed the lie that you're not good enough, declare Psalm 139:14, *"I am fearfully and wonderfully made."*
        - If you've struggled with the thought that God has abandoned you, stand on Deuteronomy 31:6, *"Be strong and of good courage, do not fear nor be afraid of them; for the Lord your God, He is the One who goes with you. He will not leave you nor forsake you."*

Session 2: Spoken Words Breed Rooted Thoughts

- Instead of saying, "I'll never be free from this struggle," declare John 8:36, *"Whom the Son sets free is free indeed."*

2. Strengthen Your Foundation:

Spend time looking up Scriptures that affirm your identity in Christ. Write them in your journal, speak them aloud, and let His truth become the foundation you stand on daily.

Here are some verses to get you started about how God defines our identity:

"But you are a chosen race, a royal priesthood, a holy nation, His own special people, that you may proclaim the praises of Him who called you out of darkness into His marvelous light;"

—1 Peter 2:9

"So God created man in his own image; in the image of God he created him; male and female He created them."

—Genesis 1:27

"I praise you for I am fearfully and wonderfully made; Marvelous are Your works, and that my soul knows very well."

—Psalm 139:14

NOTES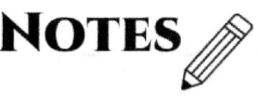

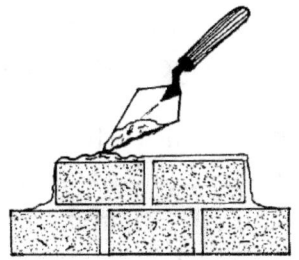

Session 3
Boundaries:
Guardrails of Grace

I stood in the kitchen, staring at the sink full of dishes, my hands clenched into fists at my sides. The house was quiet—too quiet. The kind of silence that settles after another argument. Another night of misunderstanding. Another moment of feeling unseen.

I had prayed, fasted, and done everything I thought a good wife—a good Christian wife—was supposed to do. And yet, here I was again, feeling like a stranger in my own marriage. What was it in me that kept leading me back to this place?

That question stayed with me for years, echoing in the background of my decisions, my relationships, my inner world. It took time—grace-filled time—for me to realize what I had been missing: boundaries. Not the kind built from bitterness, but the kind anchored in love. Boundaries, I would come to understand, are the

Session 3: Boundaries: Guardrails of Grace

guardrails of grace. They are not meant to keep others out, but to keep me from running off course.

I was raised in a culture where children were seen but not heard, where obedience was expected, and emotions were quietly dismissed. The unhealed trauma of my childhood didn't disappear. It followed me into adulthood, quietly shaping how I related to others. I had learned to suppress my voice, to accommodate, to make myself small in order to keep the peace. Without even realizing it, I carried that same pattern into my relationships, allowing love to mean self-sacrifice at the expense of my own well-being.

My first marriage ended when I was still young, a new mother struggling to find my footing.

My second marriage, despite my best intentions, crumbled under the weight of unspoken wounds and unhealed pain. Unfortunately, our church at the time lacked the resources to provide the guidance and support we desperately needed. I tried to be patient. I tried to love unconditionally. But I had never learned the most important thing—how to set boundaries with others and with myself.

I had mistaken sacrifice for surrender, thinking that enduring pain was a sign of faithfulness. I had believed that keeping the peace meant staying silent. But the truth was, I had never learned how to guard my heart, how to protect the woman God had created me to be.

Session 3: Boundaries: Guardrails of Grace

It wasn't until I found myself sitting in a divorce support group, listening to the stories of women who had walked similar roads, that I realized something had to change. I wasn't just healing from a broken marriage. I was healing from a broken understanding of love, especially love for myself. I had spent so many years believing that love meant losing myself for the sake of someone else. But as I sat in that room, I began to see that true love—healthy love—doesn't require you to disappear. It requires you to stand firm in who God created you to be.

The Foundation of Boundaries

Proverbs 4:23 says, *"Keep your heart with all diligence, For out of it spring the issues of life."*

I had spent years giving pieces of my heart away without guarding it. I had let my love for someone else overshadow my love for myself; and without realizing it, I had allowed relationships to define my worth instead of God.

But as I sat in that group, listening to women share their struggles, I started to understand: Boundaries weren't about building walls, which I was so good at. They were about building wisdom. They weren't about keeping people out. They were about keeping the right things in—my peace, my identity, my calling.

We all recognize physical boundaries—signs that say, "Do Not Enter," "Keep Out," or fences that mark

Session 3: Boundaries: Guardrails of Grace

where one property ends and another begins. A door that separates public space from private.

These are easy to see and understand. But emotional and relational boundaries aren't always as visible, and that's why they are often crossed without us realizing it.

Boundaries define where one person ends and another begins. They are like a fence with a door—not a solid wall—to keep the good in and the bad out. A fence provides protection, but it also has a gate, allowing access to what is healthy and life-giving while keeping out what is harmful.

Dr. Henry Cloud and Dr. John Townsend, in their book *Boundaries*, describe boundaries as knowing what is ours to control and what is not. In simple terms, boundaries define what's in my yard—my thoughts, my emotions, my choices, my responsibilities, my spiritual growth. Everything inside my yard is mine to manage; everything outside of it is not my responsibility.

For years, I had blurred these lines, feeling responsible for things that weren't mine to carry. I took on the emotional burdens of my partners, believing I could fix or change them. I tolerated unhealthy behavior because I thought setting limits would mean I wasn't loving enough.

But true love respects boundaries.

Session 3: Boundaries: Guardrails of Grace

Jesus Himself modeled this beautifully. He loved fully, yet He set clear boundaries. He walked away from crowds when He needed rest (Luke 5:16). He didn't allow people's demands to dictate His time.

He said no to distractions that pulled Him from His mission (Mark 1:38). When they wanted to make Him king, He walked away because it wasn't His mission. Jesus confronted unhealthy behavior (Matthew 23). He called out the Pharisees rather than enabling their hypocrisy.

Jesus knew His purpose, and He didn't allow guilt, manipulation, or pressure to steer Him away from God's plan. If Jesus set boundaries, then why do we feel guilty when we do the same?

Learning this truth was a turning point for me. Boundaries weren't selfish. They were necessary. They weren't about control. They were about clarity. They weren't about shutting people out. They were about letting God in.

What I Learned About Boundaries

As I walked this journey, I discovered three key lessons about boundaries.

First, I had to know my identity in Christ. Without that foundation, I couldn't discern where I ended and others began. 2 Corinthians 6:14 says, *"Do not be unequally yoked together with unbelievers. For what fellowship has righteousness with lawlessness? And*

Session 3: Boundaries: Guardrails of Grace

what communion has light with darkness?" I had assumed that if I just loved enough, prayed enough, and endured enough, things would work out. But love alone isn't enough to sustain a relationship when two people are walking in opposite directions.

Second, I learned the power of saying no. Matthew 5:37 says, *"But let your 'Yes' be 'Yes,' and your 'No,' For whatever is more than these is from the evil one."* For years, I said yes when I wanted to say no. Yes, to conversations that drained me. Yes, to obligations that left me exhausted. Yes, to relationships that required me to shrink myself. But Jesus Himself showed us the power of no. Saying no doesn't mean we are unloving—it means we are walking in wisdom.

Lastly, I knew I had to establish emotional and communication boundaries. Ephesians 4:29 says, *"Let no corrupt word proceed out of your mouth, but what is good for necessary edification, that it may impart grace to the hearers."* Instead of expecting others to read my mind, I learned to speak up. Instead of stuffing my feelings down, I expressed them with clarity and kindness. A godly marriage isn't built on silence or resentment. It's built on truth, spoken in love.

I remember the first time I truly enforced a boundary. My heart pounded as I stood my ground, unsure of how the other person would react. I had always been the one to bend, adjust, and sacrifice to

Session 3: Boundaries: Guardrails of Grace

keep the peace. But this time, something in me shifted.

I had been asked—yet again—to do something that drained me, something I had said yes to out of obligation for years. But this time, I felt God whisper, "You can say no."

And so, with my voice trembling—I did.

The response wasn't easy to hear. I was met with disappointment, confusion, and even guilt-tripping. But deep down I knew that this wasn't selfishness. It was obedience to God's call to honor the life He had given me.

When I finally embraced boundaries, something beautiful happened.

I didn't just learn how to say no—I learned how to say yes. Yes, to the kind of love that honors God. Yes, to a relationship built on respect and understanding. Yes, to a marriage where I am fully seen and known.

A God-led marriage is not built on sacrifice that erases who you are, but on mutual love, respect, and alignment with His truth. Boundaries, once seen as barriers, became the very thing that allowed me to experience the kind of relationship God had always intended for me to have.

God had a plan for my life all along. But it wasn't until I learned to set boundaries that I was truly able to

Session 3: Boundaries: Guardrails of Grace

walk in it. Jeremiah 29:11 says, *"For I know the thoughts that I think toward you, says the Lord, thoughts of peace and not of evil, to give you a future and a hope."*

And today, I live in that hope.

Closing Thoughts

Setting boundaries isn't about pushing people away—it's about creating space for God's best. At first, people may resist your boundaries, especially if they were used to you saying "yes" all the time. But remember, boundaries are an act of faith.

You are not responsible for others' reactions. You are responsible for stewarding your life, your peace, and your calling.

And in the end, when your relationships are built on healthy, God-honoring boundaries, you will find freedom, strength, and a love that is truly rooted in Jesus Christ.

Take a moment to reflect on an area of your life where you feel overwhelmed or drained. Maybe it's a relationship where you always give but rarely receive. Maybe it's an expectation that leaves you exhausted.

Step 1: Specifically identify the situation. Write down a relationship or circumstance where you struggle to say no.

Session 3: Boundaries: Guardrails of Grace

Step 2: Define your responsibility. What is yours to manage, and what is not?

Step 3: Write a boundary statement. Example: "I will no longer say yes to last-minute requests that disrupt my family time."

Step 4: Surrender it to God. Ask Him for the strength to uphold this boundary with love.

Cornerstones of Growth
- Where have I struggled with setting boundaries, and why?
- How has a lack of boundaries impacted my relationships?
- In what ways can I follow Jesus' example in setting healthier boundaries?

NOTES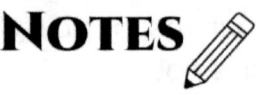

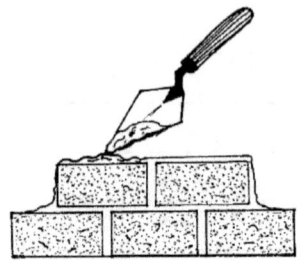

Session 4
Serving Beyond Self

"Are you going out again?" Mother stammered at me with a condemning glare.

"Yes. But only for a couple hours. No big deal." I replied. Her questioning me with that look in her eyes, as if I were committing some abominable sin just because I wanted a social life, had grown beyond annoying.

"And what about your son? You know the baby? YOUR baby I'm always taking care of?"

"Mom—don't make a big deal out of it. It's only one night."

My son slammed a spoon onto his highchair and whimpered. Mom picked him up and thrust him towards me. "YOUR baby."

I rolled my eyes. How frustrating it was every time I wanted to hang with my friends that Mom would fling

Session 4: Serving Beyond Self

a guilt trip on me. "Mom—he is fine with you. Just do what you always do. I will be back soon."

"As soon as when you walked in the door at 1:00 a.m. last week? Three nights in a row?"

"You're exaggerating again." I hated it when she always fussed at me about my social life. I was twenty-one years old and needed to be out of the house. Mom took good care of the baby. He wouldn't miss me.

She attempted to launch into a sermon, but I swiftly raised a hand in defiance, kissed my baby, and walked out the door. I was determined to have a fun night no matter what!

■■■■■■■■■■■■■■■■■■■■■■■■■■■■■■■■■

When I graduated high school, a new world opened up to me. I thought it would be a world where I could make my own decisions, come and go as I pleased, and make my own friends on my own terms. The thought of such freedom was intoxicating.

Finally an adult, at least in age, I believed that no one could tell me what to do. But what I saw as freedom proved in time to be a fragile illusion.

Beneath the surface of independence, I was subtly pulled toward choices that would bind me in other ways and lead me down roads of compromise and impulsiveness. Though still living at home and under my parents' care, in my mind, I had arrived. I believed

Session 4: Serving Beyond Self

adulthood gave me the right to do whatever I wanted, whenever I wanted. But I hadn't yet learned that real freedom comes with responsibility.

I found myself drawn into a new social scene full of parties, drinking, and drug use. Weed, cocaine, and alcohol quickly became regular companions. At the time, I didn't see them as harmful or even dangerous. I thought I was just exploring, just having fun. I wasn't intentionally trying to run from anything. I didn't even know I was running. I believed I was finally living life my way, doing the things I'd once been sheltered from.

Growing up in a Christian home, my world had been relatively safe and structured. My parents were protective and faith-filled. Church was part of life. I always knew what was expected of me. But even then, there were hints of heart rebellion beneath the surface.

I attended an all-girls high school, and some of us would sneak away during the day and walk over to the nearby boys' school. We thought we were bold and grown-up, smoking cigarettes and laughing like we didn't have a single care in the world. Nothing scandalous ever happened, but in our minds, we were pushing boundaries. Skipping class and smoking was our version of rebellion. Looking back now, I see those moments as early signs of a restless spirit: one quietly searching for freedom, attention, and maybe even love.

Session 4: Serving Beyond Self

So, when I graduated, it felt like the gates had finally opened, and I rushed through them. All the curiosity and energy I'd carried through my teenage years exploded into this season of so-called freedom. I didn't recognize it at the time, but what I thought was excitement and discovery was really a quiet ache to belong, to be seen, to be loved without conditions. I was searching for identity and purpose, but I didn't know how to find it.

I chased connection wherever I could find it—through parties, dangerous substances, and anything that made me feel noticed. On the surface, it looked like I was enjoying life. But beneath it all, I was slowly becoming more lost and disconnected from who I was created to be.

By the age of twenty-two, I had already been married and divorced and had a baby to care for. My life felt like a series of emotional crashes, broken dreams, and silent fears. I felt like parts of me were scattered in all directions, and I had no idea how to gather myself together again.

I still went to church. Maybe it was out of habit. Or maybe a quiet part of me was clinging to the thread of something familiar and holy. I sat in the pews but hadn't yet found roots in the truth I was hearing.

Even though I had a child, I didn't see myself as a mother in the fullest sense. Mind you, I loved my son with everything in me—of that there was no question. But I also craved independence, fun, and a sense of

Session 4: Serving Beyond Self

freedom that didn't match the responsibility I carried. My parents were always close by, and they adored their grandchild. That was a blessing because they helped while I worked, but I now realize it was also something I leaned on too heavily. They never said no to babysitting, and I took full advantage of that.

Sometimes, I'd go out all night, or I'd be gone the whole weekend and couldn't be reached. This was before cell phones, and understandably, my mother would grow anxious and angry. I figured, *He's in good hands.* And he was.

But what I failed to realize then is that being in good hands didn't cancel out my personal responsibility. He needed me—his mother. And, in a way, my parents did, too.

The tension between my mother and me escalated. We argued constantly. I wanted to care for my child when I was home, but she insisted she knew him better. She would complain when I wasn't there to take care of him and then complain when I was. She thought she did it better. It felt like I couldn't win. I didn't want to hear her frustration, and she didn't want to feel taken advantage of. It became a cycle of miscommunication, pride, and exhaustion on both sides.

I couldn't see it at the time, but I was living in a self-focused bubble. My desires, my freedom, my fun, my need to feel young and independent were always front and center. I told myself I was just living my life,

Session 4: Serving Beyond Self

but in doing so, I was unknowingly putting a strain on one of the most important relationships in my life: my relationship with my mother.

Then came the moment that shattered my illusion of freedom. We were in the middle of another heated argument—voices raised, emotions running high—when she said something that stopped me cold in my tracks.

"If you love your life more than your son, then maybe you should just leave. Leave him here. He's more mine than yours."

It felt like a slap! My ears burned. My stomach twisted. I was stunned, not because she was wrong, but because she was right. Her words weren't meant to punish me. They were laced with hurt, not hatred. They were spoken from the heart of a mother who had been holding everything together while watching her daughter slip away. She wasn't trying to control me. She was trying to wake me up.

And she did.

That moment marked a turning point. Something in me shifted. I couldn't ignore the truth anymore. My life wasn't just mine. It wasn't only about what I wanted, when I wanted it. I had a child, a life entrusted to me. I had a future to consider. And I had a mother who deeply loved us both, even if she didn't always say it in soft, gentle words.

Session 4: Serving Beyond Self

The shift in my habits and thinking didn't happen overnight. It was a slow and often messy process. Little by little, as I began to pull away from the destructive patterns of partying and substance use and allowed God to renew my mind, my relationship with my mother also shifted.

The more I stayed home, the more I spent time with her—not just out of necessity, but with intention. I took the time to listen to her. I chose to see her not just as my mom, but as a woman who had lived, sacrificed, and carried her own burdens. I learned to truly honor the fact that she was a woman of prayer. Her wisdom, once drowned out by my youthful defiance, resonated with me in a new way.

I saw the depth of her love, not just for me, but for my child. She had done what I hadn't yet learned to do: put someone else's needs ahead of her own. Her example stirred something in me. I knew I needed to grow up and become the mother my son deserved. That realization sparked a hunger to grow in what is called "adulting" today.

On visits to the Christian bookstore in the city, I searched for anything that could teach me how to be a better parent. I found books on motherhood, Godly parenting, and how to raise a child in the ways of the Lord. My love for reading, buried under years of chaos, awakened anew. As I poured through each book with the vigor of a true disciple, it helped me to read my Bible with fresh eyes. Scriptures that once

Session 4: Serving Beyond Self

felt distant or hard to understand came alive. They had weight. They had direction. They offered hope. And most of all, they pointed me to Jesus—the only One who could truly help me rebuild my life.

A verse that spoke directly to the change happening in me was Romans 12:1-2 NIV: *"Therefore, I urge you, brothers and sisters, in view of God's mercy, to offer your bodies as a living sacrifice, holy and pleasing to God—this is your true and proper worship. Do not conform to the pattern of this world but be transformed by the renewing of your mind in Christ Jesus, so you can prove what is the good, and perfect, and acceptable will of God."*

That Scripture felt like it was written just for me. My mother had been modeling what it meant to live sacrificially all along, offering her time, energy, and even her heart to raise my son when I wouldn't. She wasn't perfect, but she was consistent. And through her, I saw that I had been conforming to a world that told me freedom was doing whatever I wanted, whenever I wanted.

But true, transformative freedom is only found in God and comes through heart surrender—as a living sacrifice, holy and pleasing to Him. Only that would be my true and proper worship. Not just attending church when my heart was so far from Him. I needed to let God lead every part of me so that I truly would be a reflection of all His good, all His perfection, and all things acceptable to His holiness. And in my life at

Session 4: Serving Beyond Self

that time, that required me to be transformed by renewing my mind as a responsible mother to my precious little boy.

As I leaned into this truth, I was drawn to another verse that anchored my understanding of love: *"Greater love has no one than this: to lay down one's life for one's friends."* John 15:13 NIV.

That's the kind of love Jesus displayed. He had every reason to stay in heaven, yet He came down to earth to serve. He gave His life, not for Himself, but for us. He valued our redemption over His own comfort. He didn't live a self-centered life. He lived a sacrificial life. As I reflected on Jesus's sacrifice, I couldn't help but think of the Father's love, too. God the Father willingly gave His only Son for us in order to restore the broken relationship between God and mankind. Between God and . . . me!

That kind of sacrifice is unimaginable.

As a parent, I began to understand the depth of pain and love involved in that decision. Jesus didn't just come to earth by His own initiative. He obeyed the Father's will. He followed the plan, knowing the cost. The Father spoke, and the Son obeyed. That is divine love. That is sacrificial love. And it was for—me.

It was for—you.

For all of us who would choose to believe.

Session 4: Serving Beyond Self

That was the kind of love I wanted to learn to live. And that was the kind of love I wanted to give my son.

Little by little, as I leaned into Jesus, He reshaped me from the inside out. My destructive and self-centered habits didn't disappear overnight, and the struggles didn't vanish immediately. My so-called friends continued to call and invite me out. The temptation to step back into the life I had left behind still had a power to intrigue me. I wrestled with the tension of wanting to belong to that life and wanting to grow in my new life in Christ.

Something inside me had changed. I wasn't tossed about on chaotic, worldly waves anymore. I had an anchor in my faith as never before. I had direction. And I knew I couldn't move forward by going back to who I used to be.

As my heart softened, my spirit opened to God's leading, and I experienced a new kind of strength. Not the kind I used to chase through independence or survival, but the kind that comes from knowing who you belong to and why you're here.

The more I read God's Word and sat in quiet moments with Him, the more I understood that I had a purpose beyond the roles I played. I wasn't just a single mother trying to get her life together or a daughter who had disappointed her parents. I was God's daughter—redeemed, chosen, and deeply loved.

Session 4: Serving Beyond Self

Even as a little girl, I remember sitting by the window watching the neighborhood kids play basketball or handball in the playground. I didn't just see their games. I studied their faces, their body language, and the tone in their voices. I'd wonder who they were, and what their stories might be. Even then, I noticed people. Even then, I carried a seed of compassion. I just didn't know yet how God would grow it.

So, as I changed from the inside out, it wasn't a new personality that developed. It was the real me finally bursting forth. The version of me that God created me to be.

I noticed people again but this time I saw them through the eyes of Jesus. They were hurting people, lonely and lost, just like I had been. Single moms doing their best to keep going. Children craving attention and safety.

I realized this world didn't revolve around me. So many people needed love, encouragement, and support. This was the strength I was made for. Not just the strength to survive hard seasons, but the strength to pour out, to serve, to lift, and to build.

1 Peter 4:10 (ESV) states, *"Each of you should use whatever gift you have received to serve others, as faithful stewards of God's grace in its various forms."*

Session 4: Serving Beyond Self

God hard-wired me with unique strengths in showing compassion, speaking encouragement, exercising patience, and an innate ability to listen and understand the heart of others. Those gifts weren't meant to be hidden or used for personal gain. They were meant to be given away, to bless others, and to glorify God.

Serving my family, especially my son, was my first and most sacred assignment. Though not always easy, I found it no longer a burden but an offering. The more I leaned into that calling, the more I discovered joy. Not the fleeting kind I had once chased in parties and crowds, but a deep, satisfying joy that filled me with peace and purpose.

I also found new strength in serving at church. Whether helping in Sunday School, volunteering with the children's ministry, or simply showing up with a listening ear. I felt more connected to the body of Christ. I wasn't on the sidelines anymore—I was participating in something bigger than myself.

This is what spiritual health looks like. When our identity is rooted in Christ, we begin to live with purpose, powered by love and grounded in truth. We learn to move beyond ourselves, beyond our wants, our plans, and our comfort zones. We look like Jesus! We serve like Him.

True spiritual health is not just about knowing who we are in Christ, it's also about living out that identity with love, purpose, and service. When we allow Christ

Session 4: Serving Beyond Self

to transform our hearts, we shift from self-centered living to a life that reflects His sacrificial love.

Jesus didn't come to be served but to serve and give His life for others. He calls us to that same posture—not out of obligation but as an overflow of the love we've received from Him. As we humbly train our hearts and strengthen our spiritual muscles through obedience to His Word, we become carriers of God's grace in our homes, churches, and communities.

Selfless living does not mean neglecting our needs or burning ourselves out. This is not about works. Instead, it means living with intention, asking God daily, "Who can I bless today? How can I reflect Your love in this moment?" We learn to see interruptions as invitations and ordinary acts of service as sacred.

This kind of strength isn't built overnight. It's developed moment by moment, decision by decision. Every time we say no to selfishness and yes to love, we grow more spiritually healthy. We mature. We transform. And our lives begin to reflect the heart of Jesus.

You were created to live beyond yourself. To serve with joy. To shine with purpose and to glorify God with the gifts He's placed inside you. Your story, your growth, and your obedience are all part of His plan to touch the lives of others through you.

So keep showing up.

Session 4: Serving Beyond Self

Keep loving well.

Keep surrendering.

You are becoming strong in the Spirit, and that strength will last for eternity.

Cornerstones of Growth

- What personal desires or comforts have been competing with your call to love and serve others?
- How has God used a difficult truth or confrontation to help you grow spiritually?
- In what ways are you choosing to live beyond yourself right now?
- What strengths or gifts has God placed in you, and how are you using them to glorify Him?
- What spiritual disciplines can you build into your life to help you stay strong and focused on others?

Discover YOUR God-Given Strengths

You were created with a purpose. God has placed unique gifts and strengths within you—tools for serving others and glorifying Him. But sometimes, we don't recognize them right away. We question what we're good at or minimize what comes naturally to us. If you're unsure about your spiritual gifts or personal strengths, you're not alone.

Session 4: Serving Beyond Self

I wasn't always sure either. I had a sense of what came naturally, but when I took a few spiritual gifts assessments online, they gave me language and clarity that really helped. They confirmed some things I sensed and opened my eyes to gifts I hadn't fully embraced.

A Prayer for Serving Beyond Self

*Lord, thank You for the gifts you've placed in me.
Open my eyes to see them clearly,
and give me the courage to use them for your glory.
Teach me to serve others with joy and humility,
walking in the calling You designed for me.
Amen.*

BONUS: Discover Your Gifts

God has specifically designed you with gifts to serve and bless others. Sometimes those gifts are hidden until we take the time to explore them.

To support you in your journey, I've included a free online assessment to help you begin identifying the gifts God has placed in you. It's a simple, practical tool designed to help you discover how He has uniquely equipped you to serve others and walk confidently in your divine calling.

Scan QR code or visit
https://gifts.churchgrowth.org/spiritual-gifts-survey/

You are equipped.
You are called.
You are needed.

NOTES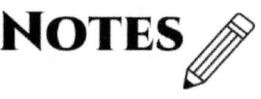

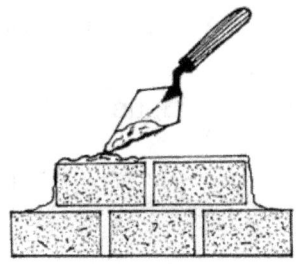

Session 5
Everyday Habits—
Eternal Impact

Every day, the stomach pain pressed a little harder, but I kept telling myself it would pass.

At work, my symptoms became harder to ignore. After watching me struggle through another afternoon shift, my employer pulled me aside with concern.

"Lillian," she said gently, "you need to see a doctor. This isn't getting better. Please. Go see a gastroenterologist and get checked out."

Reluctantly, I agreed. I scheduled an appointment and hoped for simple answers but feared what I might hear. After a series of blood tests and an uncomfortable endoscopy, I sat nervously across from the specialist and waited for his verdict. The doctor looked at me with a reassuring smile.

Session 5: Everyday Habits—Eternal Impact

"We've got some results back," he began, his tone calm but serious. "You have Celiac Disease—and you also tested positive for Lupus antibodies."

I blinked at him, my mind spinning. "Lupus I've heard of, but . . . Celiac?"

He nodded sympathetically. "Celiac Disease is an autoimmune disorder. Essentially, your body treats gluten like an enemy. Every time you eat it, your immune system attacks your small intestine. Over time, that damage can cause serious problems if it's not addressed."

He handed me a brochure with information, its pages outlining the new rules I would need to live by. "From now on," he said, "gluten is off-limits. Completely. You'll need to read every label, change how you shop, how you cook—even how you eat out. It's a big adjustment, but it's manageable. And it's essential for your health."

I nodded slowly, gripping the brochure like a lifeline. Inside, I was unraveling. How would I do this? What about dinners with my family or grabbing a quick bite with friends? Would my kitchen have to change? Would everything have to change?

Leaving the office that day, I felt like I had stepped into a new world. A world where even something as simple as a sandwich could be a hidden enemy. But deep down, I also felt a flicker of determination. If discipline was the price of health, I would learn it.

Session 5: Everyday Habits—Eternal Impact

Armed with newfound resolve, I embarked on a culinary revolution. Food labels became sacred texts on shopping trips, guiding me through a confusing labyrinth of ingredients. Once a haven of comfort, my pantry morphed overnight into a battlefield. I purged it of every gluten-laden culprit with a firm resolve to better steward my health.

The journey was especially daunting when navigating the tricky waters of eating out and social gatherings. But with God's grace, I learned to be intentional—to listen to my body's whispers and respond with care. Over time, I discovered that my physical and mental well-being were intricately tied to the nourishment I provided my body. The adage, *You are what you eat*, became a profound truth for me.

I stumbled and fell many times along the way, but my health has improved significantly since that initial diagnosis. It's a testament to the power of mindful eating, intentional routines, and unwavering determination. Learning to care for my physical body through new routines didn't happen overnight. It took patience, persistence, and a willingness to change long-held habits. It is a lifestyle I still live today.

In the same way, nurturing our spiritual health calls for daily choices to build habits that strengthen our faith. Without a steady diet of God's Word, prayer, worship, and fasting, our spirits can become just as weak and malnourished as my body once was. I've learned that if we don't tend to our souls with

Session 5: Everyday Habits—Eternal Impact

intention, we risk drifting from the very purpose and calling God has placed on our lives. Spiritual health isn't automatic. It's something we cultivate through consistent, loving discipline.

Developing Lifestyle Spiritual Habits

The same way my body needed structure and care to heal, our spirits need consistent nourishment through godly routines. Let's take a closer look at how daily disciplines shape us for the life and lifestyle God has called us to live.

Just like healing didn't come to my body through wishful thinking but through intentional practice, our spiritual health depends on what we do daily—not occasionally. Discipline might not feel glamorous, but it is the foundation of strength, and it's where transformation takes root.

We live in a world that constantly pulls us in every direction—mentally, emotionally, and spiritually. If we don't anchor ourselves in God's truth, we become vulnerable to fear, confusion, and distraction. That's why spiritual routines aren't legalistic. They're life-giving:

- They remind us of who God is.
- They reset our focus.
- They train our hearts to trust, even when life feels uncertain.

Spiritual routines aren't legalistic—
they're life-giving.

Session 5: Everyday Habits—Eternal Impact

"Train yourself toward godliness. For bodily exercise profits a little, but godliness is profitable for all things, having promise of the life that now is and of that which is to come."
—1 Timothy 4:7–8

"But solid food belongs to those who are of full age, that is, those who by reason of use have their senses exercised to discern both good and evil."
—Hebrews 5:14

In the same way, my gluten-free and dairy-free routine isn't a trend or a personal preference. It's literally lifesaving. For people with Celiac Disease, even trace amounts of gluten can trigger a severe immune response. My body mistakenly identifies gluten as a threat and attacks the lining of my small intestine, causing discomfort, inflammation, nutrient malabsorption, and lasting damage. If left unchecked, it doesn't just harm digestion—it can impair brain function, weaken the immune system, and lead to long-term neurological issues. I can't afford to be careless—not even "once in a while."

And the same is true spiritually. We can't live on occasional moments with God and expect to thrive. The world offers countless ideas, distractions, and even messages that sound good but are spiritually toxic. Like the snack aisle in a grocery store, not everything on display is nourishing. Some things may be popular or convenient, but they leave our souls starving, foggy, and spiritually inflamed. Without a daily intake of God's truth, our discernment dulls, and we can find ourselves spiritually sick without even realizing it.

You Don't Need to Start Big— You Just Need to Start

Here are core spiritual habits that will build strength over time:

Daily Time in the Word

"Man shall not live by bread alone, but by every word that proceeds from the mouth of God."
—*Matthew 4:4*

Spending daily time in God's Word is foundational to spiritual strength. The Bible is not just a book—it's our spiritual nourishment, our compass, and our sword. It teaches us who God is, who we are in Him, and how to walk in alignment with His truth.

You don't need to read several chapters a day or understand everything at once. Start right where you are. A single verse that speaks to your heart or a quiet moment meditating on a familiar passage can begin to shift everything.

Devotionals can soften the soil of your heart, but it's Scripture itself that takes root. Consider using a study Bible or concordance. A concordance helps you find Scriptures by theme, like peace, forgiveness, or strength. You can explore online resources like *Bible*

Session 5: Everyday Habits—Eternal Impact

Gateway, *Blue Letter Bible*, or even more advanced tools like *Logos Bible Software*. YouTube has many tutorials to help you get started!

The key is consistency. Whether it's a Psalm a day, a few Gospel verses, or a Bible-in-a-year plan, the Word of God will begin to shape your thoughts, renew your mind, and strengthen your spirit—one verse at a time. Even when it feels dry or ordinary, you're sowing seeds that will bear fruit.

Prayer

Prayer is one of our most powerful spiritual disciplines—and often one of the most misunderstood. Many of us treat it like a one-way conversation. But prayer is meant to be two-way. It's not just presenting needs; it's pausing to hear what's on God's heart.

Think of prayer like a relationship. If every conversation you had with someone was one-sided, that relationship would feel shallow. It's the same with God. He longs to hear from us but also wants us to listen.

Prayer isn't limited to a few quiet minutes—it's a continual awareness of God's presence. Whether I'm driving, cleaning, or in conversation, I've learned to talk to Jesus in the middle of it all. It's not about completing a checklist. It's about staying in communion with the One who knows and loves me best.

Session 5: Everyday Habits—Eternal Impact

Worship

Some of my most meaningful worship experiences have come in quiet places—folding laundry, cleaning, or simply sitting in stillness. Worship isn't confined to Sunday mornings; it happens when we live aware of God's goodness and respond with gratitude.

One of my personal go-to songs is *It Is Well with My Soul*. No matter what kind of day I'm having, that hymn centers me. It reminds me that peace doesn't come from perfect circumstances but from God's presence.

The hymn was written by Horatio Spafford after the tragic loss of his four daughters at sea. As his ship neared the site of their death, he penned the lyrics: *"When peace like a river attendeth my way, when sorrows like sea billows roll..."* Even through heartbreak, he chose worship. That kind of faith humbles me. Worship is often born from surrender, not ease.

Fasting

You can begin with skipping a meal or even taking a day off from social media. Fasting humbles the body and tunes the heart. It reminds us that we don't live on bread alone but on every word from God (Matthew 4:4).

Fasting has helped me reset when I felt spiritually dry or confused. Whether fasting from food, entertainment, or even certain conversations, the goal

Session 5: Everyday Habits—Eternal Impact

isn't deprivation—it's deeper dependence on God. It says, "God, You are my source—not this thing I'm letting go of."

It's not always easy. It may bring discomfort, but those moments become invitations to lean in. Every time we fast with the right heart, God meets us powerfully.

We often expect growth to be a straight line, but it rarely is. There are days I knowingly ate something with gluten—and paid the price. And spiritually, I sometimes skip my devotions or lose focus in prayer. But the journey toward discipline isn't about being flawless—it's about being faithful.

But the journey toward discipline isn't about being flawless—it's about being faithful.

God isn't looking for perfect routines. He's looking for a heart that keeps returning to Him. When you fall off track, don't let shame keep you stuck. Let grace draw you back. Just like I learned to get back up, drink water, rest, and reset my diet after a flare-up—we must do the same spiritually. Rest in God's grace. Reset your focus. Start again.

"And let us not grow weary while doing good, for in due season we shall reap if we do not lose heart."
—Galatians 6:9

God isn't building spiritual strength in us just for our benefit—He's preparing us to carry something

Session 5: Everyday Habits—Eternal Impact

eternal. When we're spiritually strong, we can walk boldly in our calling, serve others with compassion, and persevere through trials. Our daily disciplines don't just shape us—they shape our legacy.

Your routine isn't just shaping your day— it's shaping your legacy.

Cornerstones of Growth

Take a moment to reflect on the spiritual practices shared in this chapter. These questions are designed to help you apply what you've read and strengthen your walk with God—one step at a time.

- **Daily Time in the Word:**
  What is one small, consistent step you can take to build or strengthen your daily time in God's Word this week?

- **Worship:**
  What helps you shift your focus from yourself to God in worship—and how can you create more space for that in your daily life?

- **Prayer:**
  When do you feel most connected to God in prayer—when you're talking, listening, journaling, or simply being still?

- **Fasting:**
  What distractions or comforts might God be

Session 5: Everyday Habits—Eternal Impact

inviting you to surrender—temporarily or regularly—so you can draw closer to Him?

Spiritual strength isn't built in a day—it's built day by day. Some moments will feel powerful; others may feel quiet or difficult. But every time you choose to open your Bible, whisper a prayer, offer praise, or fast from something for the sake of intimacy with God, you are training your spirit to trust Him more.

Keep showing up. He's meeting you there.

"The Lord is near to all who call upon Him, to all who call upon Him in truth."
—Psalm 145:18

NOTES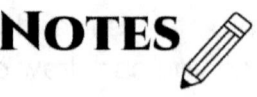

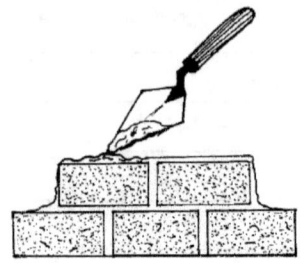

Session 6
Vision Born from Purpose

Around 2017, I sensed a deeper call to step into more of what God had planned for me.

That same year, I completed my bachelor's degree in behavioral science with a minor in child advocacy. I was fifty-nine years old and felt proud—not just of the diploma but of the journey it represented. Age is never a barrier when it comes to learning, growing, or walking in obedience to God's call. Every season of life can be a launching point when God is leading.

A few years after graduating, a friend introduced me to the author Valorie Burton. As I read her work and explored more about her background, I learned that she had launched a coaching organization called The CaPP Institute (Coaching and Positive Psychology). The idea of coaching immediately captured my attention. Over several days I returned to the website, read every detail, and prayed in my heart, *Lord, is this something You're leading me to?*

Session 6: Vision Born from Purpose

It was time to share with my husband what was on my mind and heart. "I think this might be the next step for me," I said. "It lines up with everything I've been learning, and it just seems right."

He listened carefully, asked thoughtful questions and said, "This sounds like something you were made for. What do you want to do?"

"Well," I topped off his coffee and sat down beside him. "There is a three-day course available in Peachtree, Georgia I'd like to go to. I could get my certification as a life coach. What do you think?" I entrusted this decision to the Lord leading through my husband.

To my delight and deep gratitude, my husband offered to cover the cost of the trip and the coaching program. His enthusiastic support reminded me of how powerful it is when a husband and wife walk together in unity. Centered in God's will, how beautifully God weaves purpose and partnership together.

That weekend in Georgia changed everything. It was one of the first times I saw a real path forward—not just in what I could do, but in who I was becoming. It felt like a door had opened to the next season of my life.

Although the course itself was just three days, it was packed with intensive training, rich content, and hands-on learning. I later completed the full requirements to earn my coaching certification through the CaPP Institute, which further deepened both my skills and my calling.

After earning my certification, I started my coaching career one-on-one with a few individuals. These were faith-based sessions where prayer, scripture, and spiritual encouragement were naturally woven into each conversation. Because my coaching always included my faith, I knew I wanted to grow more deeply in that area of faith-based coaching, both spiritually and professionally.

I pursued and later received my certification as a Christian Life Coach through Light University. This additional training gave me even greater clarity and spiritual depth in how to equip others to live with intention, faith, and spiritual strength. God wasn't just allowing me to dream—He was refining my vision to align with His Kingdom.

Lifting Our Eyes First

We all want clarity in life—especially when it comes to our calling. But clarity doesn't begin with a vision board or goal list. It begins with purpose. Direction flows from purpose. It's not something we invent but something God reveals as we align our lives with His divine assignment for us.

This session is about discovering the connection between your God-given purpose and the picture in your mind that flows from it. Vision that's born from

Session 6: Vision Born from Purpose

purpose is tied to destiny—it brings fulfillment, clarity, and direction. But when we create vision apart from purpose, it can leave us feeling restless and frustrated. We must explore how to recognize purpose, clarify the images you see, and create a faith-filled vision board rooted in God's will.

I've always believed in the power of purpose and vision. Among the many things I'm learning on this journey is that if I'm not placing my purpose and vision in God's hands first, surrendering them to His will, they can quickly lead me off track. It's so easy to get laser-focused on the dream, the plan, the next step and forget to look up. I've had moments when I was so locked in on what was ahead of me that I lost sight of the One who sees the whole picture.

God's view is higher. His wisdom is greater, and His timing is perfect. While I'm looking at the here and now, He's already in tomorrow. But when I stop trying to control everything and fix my eyes on Him, that's when true peace and direction come. His plan will always be better than mine, and His power has no limits.

"For My thoughts are not your thoughts, nor are your ways My ways," says the Lord. "For as the heavens are higher than the earth, so are My ways higher than your ways, and My thoughts than your thoughts."
—Isaiah 55:8–9

Session 6: Vision Born from Purpose

From Purpose to Vision

When God realigned my life, He didn't just give me a new path—He gave me purpose. And out of that purpose, vision was born.

Clarity is the visual reality of your purpose. It's recognizing what you were born to do, the perception of your divine assignment. Vision is not something you invent. It's something revealed.

When vision is rooted in purpose, it aligns with your destiny. But when it's based solely on personal ambition or desire, it often leads to frustration, not fulfillment.

Insight comes when your past experiences collide with your present and begin shaping your future.

It's seeing beyond what your eyes can see—into the imagination of faith.

And here's the shocker: Vision is not just all about you. It is meant to benefit others. That's why purpose and a clear focus need perspective. Your training, your preparation, even your past, are all elements God uses to bring about His good will and purposes for your life. Though He does not cause the ill and painful things that may have happened to you, He redeems what the enemy meant for evil and makes them work for your ultimate good in Him—His vision, purpose, and destiny for your life.

Session 6: Vision Born from Purpose

"And we know that all things work together for good to those who love God, to those who are the called according to His purpose."

—Romans 8:28

Purpose is the divine assignment of your life—why you're here, what you were born for, as noted in the book of Esther 4:14, "for such a time as this."

For a number of years, I have studied and taught the effectiveness of vision boards—not as a shortcut to success, but as a faith-filled tool to reflect what God has taught me. I led workshops and helped others pause, reflect, and seek God's direction before setting vision. These sessions became sacred spaces where people rediscovered their "why" and embraced God's dreams over their own.

When we see our purpose clearly, vision becomes something we can respond to with faith and action. When guided by the Holy Spirit and aligned with Scripture, it's not about crafting a perfect collage display. It's about creating a place of focus, encouragement, and faithful expectation in a visual reminder of the dreams and direction God is birthing in your heart.

Create a God-Centered Vision Board

Pause and Pray

Before you begin, pause and make space for God. Spend time in prayer asking Him to reveal His heart

Session 6: Vision Born from Purpose

for your life. Invite the Holy Spirit to search your heart and clarify what matters most. Let this be a quiet, unhurried time of listening and surrender.

Ask God to bring to the surface any hidden desires, buried dreams, or divine assignments that may be waiting to be rediscovered. Psalm 37:4 reminds us: *"Delight yourself also in the Lord, and He shall give you the desires of your heart."*

As you delight in Him, trust that the desires stirring in your heart are not random—they are significant and seen by God. Whether it's the desire to write, sing, start a business, get married, have a baby, or step into ministry, bring it to Him in prayer. This is where vision begins—with an open heart and a surrendered spirit.

Remember, God is not limited by what we see or imagine—*"Now to Him who is able to do exceedingly abundantly above all that we ask or think . . ."* Ephesians 3:20.

Put It on Paper

As you spend time praying and reflecting, write down what God has placed on your heart. Journaling brings clarity and helps you stay focused when distractions arise.

Think through key areas of your life—faith, family, health, finances, relationships, calling, ministry, and personal growth. What is God calling you to pursue in this season?

Session 6: Vision Born from Purpose

This is the time to engage your imagination muscle. What dreams have been stirring within you? Capture them in writing. As you do, you're not just making a list—you're acknowledging the seeds of vision God may be planting.

Keep in mind the instruction from *"Write the vision; make it plain on tablets, so he may run who reads it. For still the vision awaits its appointed time . . . If it seems slow, wait for it; it will surely come; it will not delay"* Habakkuk 2:2–3 (ESV). God honors us when we take the time to write down the vision He's given us.

Gather Supplies
You'll need:
- A poster board or cork board
- Magazines, downloaded or printed words or images, scissors, glue/tape
- Bible verses, quotes, or affirmations that speak to your purpose
- Markers or stickers for added personalization as you please
- Comfortable place to work with tea/coffee and treats by your side
- A relaxing playlist to provide a thoughtful ambience

A. Create a Visual Reflection of Purpose Look through the magazines for images and words that resonate with what God has placed on your heart—not just what looks pretty or trendy. Select items that

Session 6: Vision Born from Purpose

represent values, promises, or future direction rooted in faith. Find exact images or words through an online search and print out as needed.
- Copy, paste, and print free images online through Google Images, Pixaby, Splash, Canva, or other websites.
- Type out key words in varied sizes and fonts using your Word documents. Print and cut.

B. Assemble Your Board Arrange the images and words in a way that brings clarity and inspiration. You might group items by category or theme. Include a Scripture in the center or top as a spiritual anchor.

C. Display and Declare Place your board somewhere you'll see it often—your prayer corner, office, or bedroom. Use it as a reminder to speak life, stay focused, and trust God's timing.

D. Revisit Regularly Review your board throughout the year. Let it be a place of thanksgiving as you witness God's faithfulness, and a prompt for prayer when facing obstacles.

Remember: Your vision board isn't about perfection. It's about perspective. It's a visual altar that helps you remain anchored in God's promises while moving forward in faith.

Session 6: Vision Born from Purpose

Cornerstones of Growth

- Have you ever pursued a vision that wasn't tied to your purpose? What did you learn from that experience?
- In what areas of your life is God inviting you to shift your perspective and look up—to lift your eyes from your plans and fix them on Him?
- Before creating a vision board or writing your purpose statement, take time to pray: "God, show me what You see. Align my heart and purpose with Your will."
- Reflect on your past: What key life experiences, challenges, or victories do you believe God has used to shape your purpose?
- Write a personal purpose statement—your life mission statement—that summarizes what you believe God has called you to in this season. Keep it short, prayerful, and rooted in Scripture.

Example: "I help (who?) women (do what?) build lives that are spiritually strong and built to last—(how?) grounded in God's truth, purpose, and daily practice."

NOTES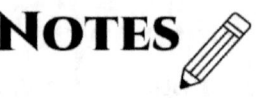

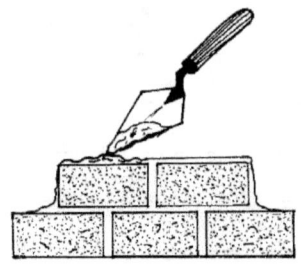

Session 7
A Grateful Heart

Personal Reflection:
His Goodness in My Story

As I reflect on my life's journey, I give God all the glory for how He's restored what once felt broken. Looking back on the losses, the victories, the pain, and the healing, I can see how God used it all.

Even when I didn't understand, even when I resisted, He was shaping me. Molding me. Preparing me. And when I finally surrendered, I realized that nothing was wasted. Every tear, every heartache, every lesson worked together for a greater purpose.

Today, I stand in awe of what God has done. I am grateful not just for what He's brought me through but for who I've grown into because of Him. My past became part of my purpose. The hard places became life lessons I now live by. And my testimony is a

Session 7: A Grateful Heart

constant reminder that God will always take what is meant to break me and mold it into that which will build me.

One of the greatest blessings in my life is the incredible man God brought into my world—a man of character, a man after God's own heart. He stepped in and stepped up to help raise my four children with love, strength, and integrity. That kind of grace doesn't just happen. It's God.

Now those four children are grown, many with children of their own. And I have the joy of being a grandmother—what I believe is one of the greatest callings on earth. There's something sacred about seeing the fruit of your prayers and sacrifices reflected in the next generation. I don't take any of it for granted.

Today, I'm using the experiences of my past, both the painful and the beautiful, to sow seeds of hope into the lives of other women. After almost six decades, I'm still learning. Still growing. Still discovering new depths of God's grace and mercy.

His mercies truly are new every morning.

And now, as I write this book, it humbles me. It overwhelms me. Not because I think I have all the answers, but because I know what it means to be rescued by God, to be rebuilt by Him, and to be used by Him despite my flaws.

Session 7: A Grateful Heart

That's the joy and peace I carry. A peace that truly surpasses all understanding. (Philippians 4:7) It's not pride. It's praise. And it's all for His glory.

Gratitude shifts everything. It reminds us that we are not alone and that God's hand has been on us all along—even in the hard places. But we must never take His goodness for granted.

As we come to the end of this spiritual training journey together, I want to invite you to step back and look at the full picture of what each session has challenged you with.

Imagine building a great tower of strength, purpose, and impact. Each chapter session can be likened to a brick—carefully placed, purposefully aligned. One by one, these spiritual bricks helped to build something strong. Something lasting. Something that points upward, soaring towards heaven. A life built to last.

We laid our brick foundation with identity and forgiveness, learning who we are in Christ and releasing the weight of past hurts.

Then we added the power of words—bricks that recognize how what we speak and hear shapes our lives.

We laid out boundaries, understanding when to say yes and when to say no with Godly wisdom.

Session 7: A Grateful Heart

We expanded upward into serving beyond self. There we learned the strength of sacrificial love and our call to pour into others.

The building blocks of discipline reminded us that spiritual strength requires consistency and alignment. Not perfection, but daily intention.

As we rose higher, we could see with purpose where we recognized and embraced our God-given assignments.

And now—gratitude. Not just the final brick, but the mortar that binds all these bricks together. Gratitude keeps us grounded. It opens our eyes and our hearts. It strengthens our spirit and honors the heart of God.

When you pick up your trowel/pen, dip it into mortar-ink, and bind the bricks of your day with gratitude your mind is renewed. Be intentional to journal your tower-growth. Stop at the end of the day, or even first thing in the morning, and record your thoughts. What went right today? What was good about yesterday?

Scientists have found that our brains are wired to notice the negative first. It's a survival instinct, but often leaves us feeling depleted and discouraged. That's why we must train ourselves to focus on the good. On God's goodness.

Just journaling your gratitude daily has been shown to improve sleep, lower stress, strengthen self-

Session 7: A Grateful Heart

esteem, and lead to healthier habits. It can even deepen your connection with others—and with God.

Journal one thing you're thankful for every day for the next thirty days. It doesn't have to be deep or dramatic. Just be honest. Be intentional. Watch how your spirit begins to lift, and your perspective starts to change.

Because here's the truth:
Gratitude invites God's power
into your situation.

A brick in my life where my heart overflows with gratitude is in God's provision.

He has always been my provider—especially during my single years raising four children on my own. Looking back, I saw His hand on us over and over again. Yes, I'm grateful for the steady jobs He blessed me with, work that allowed me to provide for my family. That was His grace.

But His provision went far beyond a paycheck. He spared me from many costs I never had to bear, like medical bills or emergencies. Our home never suffered major damage, and it was never broken into. I never had to face a catastrophic accident that would have left me unable to work. My car was never stolen, and I rarely had to deal with expensive repairs. These are the quiet mercies we often overlook. But they are part of God's provision too.

Session 7: A Grateful Heart

Then there were the gifts in kind: groceries that showed up just when we needed them, money or gift cards tucked into envelopes from friends or family, hand-me-down clothes, especially for the girls. Support came through people God placed in our lives. His generosity wasn't always wrapped in cash. It often came through kindness.

I've come to see that God's provision is layered. He provides through earnings, yes—but also through what He protects us from and how He provides through others. His economy is full of unseen savings, unexpected gifts, and everyday miracles.

All these things I recorded in my journal. God was faithful in my yesterdays, and I still see His faithfulness today. He continues to take care of me. Still faithful. Still providing.

The Power of Gratitude in Daily Life

If you want to shift your entire outlook on life—from the negative to the positive—focus on gratitude. It's one of the most powerful ways to move into a place of peace and joy, no matter what's happening around you. As a life coach, I've seen it again and again: gratitude is the key that unlocks all doors to daily strength, personal purpose, and lifestyle impact:

- Gratitude leads to greater happiness, stronger relationships, and better health.
- Gratitude clears your progress toward goals and builds determination.

Session 7: A Grateful Heart

- Gratitude inspires generosity, improves sleep, and boosts self-esteem.
- Gratitude fixes our thoughts on what is good and godly. A thankful heart sharpens our spiritual vision and helps us see life through the lens of God's faithfulness.

There's truly no downside to practicing gratitude. God designed our hearts to be drawn to what we focus on. When we choose to give thanks, we see more of His goodness in our everyday lives. The Apostle Paul reminds us of this in Philippians 4:8: *"Finally, brethren, whatever things are true, whatever things are noble, whatever things are just, whatever things are pure, whatever things are lovely, whatever things are of good report, if there is any virtue and if there is anything praiseworthy—meditate on these things."*

God has done so much in my life that I've often found myself overwhelmed in the best ways. If I only focused on the disappointments in my past, I would have ended up stuck in a place of grief. But gratitude lifted my spirit from the dungeon to the high tower of His strength, purpose, and life impact.

That's one of the reasons I journal. Looking back, I can trace His fingerprints—see the doors He opened, the storms He calmed, the strength He gave me to stand. It's my reminder that if He did it before, He'll do it again.

Session 7: A Grateful Heart

Magnify what God has done in your life. Don't just think about it—write it down.

Let gratitude anchor your thoughts and shape your perspective. Don't forget the big picture of what He's already done because you focus on what hasn't happened yet. Focus on the good that is happening, even if it's small. Psalm 100 reminds us to *"Enter into His gates with thanksgiving, and into His courts with praise. Be thankful and bless His name."*

So, keep building. Keep showing up with a grateful heart. Because when you do, you're not just surviving—you're becoming strong, steady, and unshakable. You're becoming someone whose life is truly built to last.

Cornerstones of Growth

- List some ways you've seen God provide—not just financially, but through protection, relationships, or unexpected kindness?
- When was the last time you thanked God for who He is, not just for what He's done?
- In what areas of your life do you need to refocus on gratitude instead of disappointment?
- What would change if you started journaling about one thing you're thankful for every day?

NOTES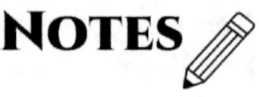

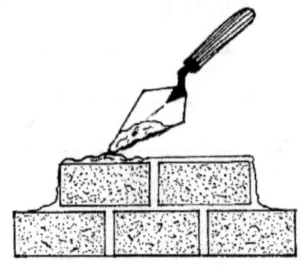

Post-Assessment: How Have You Grown?

Now in my senior years, I find deep solace in reflecting on my journey with Jesus—over four decades of His faithfulness.

As I look back with a grateful heart, I see countless moments when God pulled me from the depths—some trials brought on by life's hardships and others by my own choices. In those dark seasons, when I had nothing left but a desperate cry—"Help me, Lord"—God was faithful. Every single time, He answered.

He didn't cause my struggles, but He never wasted them. What the enemy meant for harm, God turned for my good. (Genesis 50:20)

Through the years, I've discovered unshakable spiritual principles that have nourished my soul and kept my faith strong. As paradoxical as it may seem, I am grateful for the challenges I have faced. The pain of childhood molestation, the heartache of failed

Post-Assessment: How Have You Grown?

relationships, and the weight of health struggles could have left me broken. Instead, they became the very experiences that shaped me. They led me deeper into faith, built resilience within me, gave me a new identity, and refined my purpose—to serve God and strengthen others.

Looking back, I don't just see struggles anymore; I see the hand of a loving Father who has been with me every step of the way. And for that, I am forever grateful.

Now that you've completed *Built to Last*, take a moment to revisit the questions from the Pre-Assessment. Use the same 1–5 scale to reflect honestly on your growth. Journal your answers, compare where you started, and celebrate the progress—no matter how small. This is your journey of spiritual strength.

1 = Not at all   2 = Rarely   3 = Sometimes
4 = Often   5 = Consistently

Self-Reflection & Spiritual Awareness

I take time to reflect on my life and my walk with God.
Answer: _____

I seek God's perspective on my circumstances rather than reacting based on my emotions.
Answer: _____

Post-Assessment: How Have You Grown?

I regularly spend time in prayer and the Word of God. Answer: _____

Identifying Areas for Growth

I am aware of the spiritual areas in my life that need strengthening. Answer: _____

I take intentional steps to renew my mind and align my thoughts with God's truth. Answer: _____

I recognize and challenge negative thoughts that do not align with God's promises. Answer: _____

Embracing Self-Discipline

I maintain a consistent spiritual practice (e.g., prayer, worship, Bible study). Answer: _____

I follow through on spiritual commitments, even when I don't feel like it. Answer: _____

I set aside distractions and make time to be still before God. Answer: _____

Discovering God's Unique Assignment

I have a sense of God's purpose for my life. Answer: _____

I use my gifts and talents in ways that honor God and serve others. Answer: _____

Post-Assessment: How Have You Grown?

I trust God's timing and direction, even when I don't have all the answers. Answer: _____

Final Reflection—Open-Ended Questions
Write your responses in your journal:
- What new habits have you developed?
- What truths have taken root in your heart? How would you describe your current level of spiritual strength?
- How has your perspective shifted? Where do you sense God is inviting you to grow next?

Spiritual growth is a journey—not a destination. As you look back on your transformation, remember that every step you've taken has drawn you closer to God's purpose for your life's assignment.

Use this time of reflection as a reminder that God is continually working in you, strengthening your spirit, and shaping you for His greater plan.

I'd love to hear how this book has enriched your life. Feel free to reach out at:

mrslillianbaker@gmail.com

Be Blessed and Be a Blessing!

Final Blessing

May your heart remain soft with gratitude, no matter the season.

May you never forget the goodness of God in your life—His provision, His protection, His presence.

May you continue to build a life of spiritual strength, one decision, one prayer, one act of love at a time.

And may the Tower of Faith you are building rise strong, purposeful, and impact your world, pointing to the One who made you and sustains you.

Let your identity be rooted in Christ,
Your words be filled with power,
Your boundaries be guided by wisdom,
Your love be poured out in service,
Your discipline be anchored in grace,
Your vision be set by heaven,
And your gratitude be constant and contagious.

You are truly "Built to Last."
Be blessed and be a blessing.

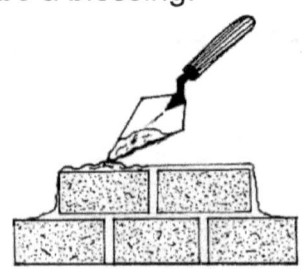

About the Author

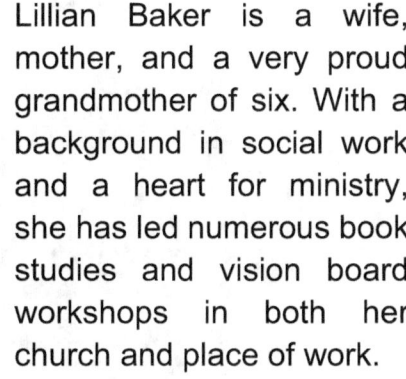

Lillian Baker is a wife, mother, and a very proud grandmother of six. With a background in social work and a heart for ministry, she has led numerous book studies and vision board workshops in both her church and place of work.

Lillian holds a Bachelor's Degree in Behavioral Science from Wilmington University, a Life Coach Certificate from the Coaching and Positive Psychology Institute (CaPP), and a Christian Life Coach Certificate from Light University of the American Association of Christian Counselors. She has also contributed devotionals to *The Secret Place* booklets.

As a certified Christian life coach, Lillian is passionate about equipping women to grow stronger in faith, embrace their God-given identity, and complete their unique assignments (John 17:4 MSG). Her book, *Built to Last: A Spiritual Training Guide for Strength, Purpose, and Impact* invites readers to build unshakable spiritual foundations that can withstand every season of life. Connect with Lillian at www.lillianbaker.com.

About Pageant Wagon Publishing

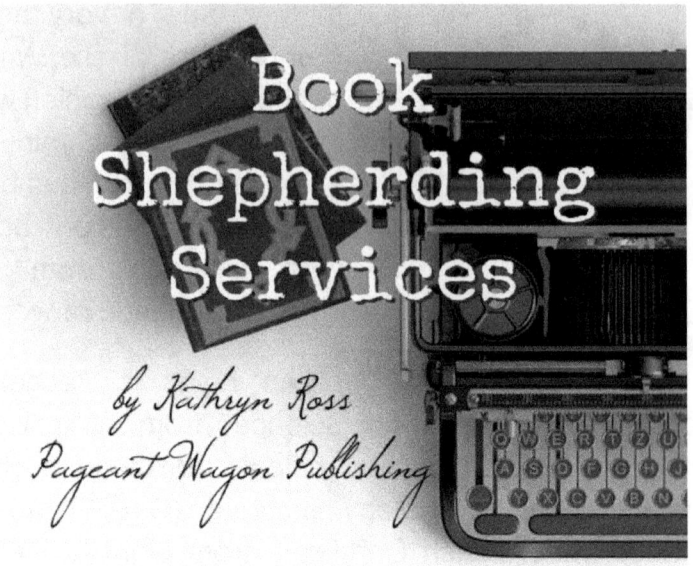

Let me help you develop the book God is calling you to write ~
From Idea to Finished Product!

A la carte and bundle services include:
~ Monthly Consulting Sessions
~ Editing
~ Layout & Design
~ Print Publishing
~Audio Book Recording
~ Ghostwriting

www.pageantwagonpublishing.com
info@pageantwagonpublishing.com

www.ingramcontent.com/pod-product-compliance
Lightning Source LLC
LaVergne TN
LVHW051526070426
835507LV00023B/3330